Sérgio Éberson da Silva Maia
Thiago Fonseca Silva
Jefferson D. M. de Matos

Clinical and epidemiological profile of injuries to the maxillofacial complex

Sérgio Éberson da Silva Maia
Thiago Fonseca Silva
Jefferson D. M. de Matos

Clinical and epidemiological profile of injuries to the maxillofacial complex

Etiology, Classification and Management

ScienciaScripts

Imprint

Any brand names and product names mentioned in this book are subject to trademark, brand or patent protection and are trademarks or registered trademarks of their respective holders. The use of brand names, product names, common names, trade names, product descriptions etc. even without a particular marking in this work is in no way to be construed to mean that such names may be regarded as unrestricted in respect of trademark and brand protection legislation and could thus be used by anyone.

Cover image: www.ingimage.com

This book is a translation from the original published under ISBN 978-613-9-65503-8.

Publisher:
Sciencia Scripts
is a trademark of
Dodo Books Indian Ocean Ltd. and OmniScriptum S.R.L publishing group

120 High Road, East Finchley, London, N2 9ED, United Kingdom
Str. Armeneasca 28/1, office 1, Chisinau MD-2012, Republic of Moldova, Europe
Printed at: see last page
ISBN: 978-620-7-42074-2

SERGIO EBERSON DA SILVA MAIA

CLINICAL AND EPIDEMIOLOGICAL PROFILE OF PATIENTS WITH INJURIES TO THE MAXILLOFACIAL COMPLEX

Authors:

Sergio Eberson da Silva Maia

Dental Surgeon - graduated from Centro Universitario Doutor Leao Sampaio, UNILEAO, Juazeiro do Norte - CE.

Resident of the Oral and Maxillofacial Surgery and Traumatology Program at the UFPI University Hospital, Teresina - PI.

Thiago Fonseca Silva

Dental Surgeon - graduated from the State University of Montes Claros, UNIMONTES, MG.

Specialist in Orthodontics at the Modal Institute in Belo Horizonte, MG.

Master's degree from the State University of Montes Claros, UNIMONTES, MG.

PhD in Molecular Medicine from the Federal University of Minas Gerais, UFMG.

Adjunct Professor of Orthodontics, Department of Dentistry, Universidade Federal dos Vales do Jequitinhonha e Mucuri - UFVJM, Diamantina - MG.

Anyelen Remigio de Gois

Dental Surgery - graduated from Centro Universitario Doutor Leao Sampaio, UNILEAO, Juazeiro do Norte - CE.

Postgraduate student in Minor Oral Surgery ABO - Petrolina - PE.

Matheus Inacio de Lima

Dental Surgeon - graduated from Centro Universitario Doutor Leao Sampaio,

UNILEAO, Juazeiro do Norte - CE.

Postgraduate student in Orthodontics

Alerico Dias Vieira

Dental Surgeon - graduated from Centro Universitario Doutor Leao Sampaio, UNILEAO, Juazeiro do Norte - CE.

Postgraduate student in Orthodontics

Jefferson David Melo de Matos

Dental Surgeon - graduated from Centro Universitario Doutor Leao Sampaio, UNILEAO, Juazeiro do Norte - CE.

Master's student in the Post-Graduation Program in Restorative Dentistry - Specialty in Dental Prosthesis at Universidade Estadual Paulista Julio Mesquita Filho (UNESP - Sao Jose dos Campos).

Address for correspondence

Rua 31 de margo, n 2457, Bairro Ininga - Teresina - PI

Apartment 302, block B

Email: sergioeberson@gmail .com

PREFACE

This project presents a summary of the research carried out over the course of five years of my undergraduate degree in dentistry. It is intended to serve as support material for academics and clinical professionals who, like me, are passionate about oral and maxillofacial surgery and trauma, especially with regard to the care of patients with facial trauma and injuries to the soft tissues of the maxillofacial region. This material is based on research carried out in a hospital environment, based on a retrospective analysis of cases of patients who had injuries to the maxillofacial complex, with the aim of verifying the main etiological factors, as well as the architecture of these injuries, their location and the treatment used. The other part consists of a literature review, which consulted scientific articles and works by renowned authors and references for Oral and Maxillofacial Surgery, such as Miloro, Fonseca, Hupp, Prado, among others. It is worth emphasizing that this work does not exclude the importance of reading these works, especially for those who wish to deepen their knowledge in the management of these lesions, however the material provides a compilation of up-to-date information on this subject which is little explored.

Sergio Eberson S. Maia.

DEDICATION

I dedicate this work to my wife Andreia Alencar, who has always been by my side and without her support, love and dedication I would never have achieved this victory, and to my daughter Livia Marilis, an angel that God placed in my care, who fills my life with joy. First of all, I would like to thank God who has enlightened my path throughout this journey, my father Edilson de Oliveira, my mother Maria Zilda and my brothers Samuel, Santiago, Sara and Sales and my grandmother Maria do Socorro who have always supported and encouraged me on this journey. To my teacher Thiago Fonseca Silva for his patience in guiding and encouraging me to complete this work. To all the teachers on the course, who have been so important in my academic life. I would like to dedicate this to my college friends and colleagues, for their constant encouragement and support, and to my long-time friends Roberto, Francisco and Cristiano, who, even though they are far away, are rooting for my success. I would also like to thank my work colleagues at the HMMV in Trindade and the HRJL in Picos for their encouragement. I would also like to thank my friends Josenildo Gomes and Ednaldo Souza for their advice and support in difficult decisions, and my first teachers Fabio Gomes and Drummond Stenio, who were great encouragers of my personal and professional growth, and whom I look up to as examples of perseverance and professionalism.

SUMMARY

Facial wounds come in many forms and vary in complexity. They are treated according to their extent, depth, degree of contamination, etiologic agent and exposure time. The risk of infection and unsatisfactory aesthetics are related to injuries with longer tissue exposure times. **The** aim of this study was to assess the prevalence and characteristics of soft tissue injuries in the craniofacial region in patients treated at the Maria Veneri Municipal Hospital in Trindade, Pernambuco, between June 2014 and June 2015. This study is a retrospective analysis of a sample of 213 patients. All the data was collected by analyzing the emergency room's care bulletins and the nursing team's reports. Information on personal data and the circumstances of the trauma was recorded on a specific trauma assessment form. The etiology of facial injuries was as follows: motorcycle accidents (46.9%), interpersonal violence (20.7%) and falls (10.3%). The most common types of injury were cut-contusions (42.7%), abrasions (16.9%) and lacerations (11.3%). The most affected areas were the frontal region (20.7%), the cheek (16%) and the orbital region (15.5%). Most of the cases were treated with sutures (77.5%). Motorcycle accidents are the most prevalent cause of soft tissue injuries in the facial complex. The frontal, cheek and orbital regions are the sites most commonly affected by injuries.

Keywords: Traffic accident. Soft tissue injury. Facial injuries. Facial trauma.

SUMMARY

Chapter 1   7

Chapter 2   12

Chapter 3   28

Chapter 4   33

Chapter 5   36

Chapter 6   39

CHAPTER 1.

Injuries to the maxillofacial complex

Injuries to the soft tissues of the oral and maxillofacial (BMF) complex are of great importance in the care of traumatized patients (VIEIRA *et al.,* 2013; LEITE SEGUNDO *et al.,* 2007; PETERSON, 2004). The literature describes various etiological factors related to these injuries, such as motor vehicle accidents, falls, sports-related trauma and interpersonal violence (ROSELINO *et al.,* 2009). As As a result, trauma to the soft tissues of the face can cause anything from minor abrasions and hematomas to severe blunt injuries to the skin, muscles and possibly damage to the nerves and vessels of the face (JARDIN *et al.,* 2010). The treatment of these injuries is aimed at re-establishing the function of the affected region, as well as minimizing the patient's physical sequelae (AMERICAN COLLEGE OF SURGEONS COMMITTEE ON TRAUMA - ATLS, 2004).

Soft tissue trauma of the oral and maxillofacial region is a common clinical situation in the daily life of emergency units and hospitals, especially in large urban centers and in regions with an increased demand for mobility, associated with traffic violations and growing levels of crime (SASTRY *et al.,* 1995).

According to the World Health Organization (WHO), facial trauma is among the main causes of morbidity and mortality, affecting the population with great epidemiological variability, without distinguishing between age, gender, income or geographical location. Facial injuries represent a significant injury in world health and have a high incidence and diversity in form and severity (KRUG *et al.,* 2000). Soft tissue trauma in the oral and maxillofacial region comes in many forms and varies in complexity, and is dealt with according to its extent, depth, degree of contamination, etiologic agent and exposure time (SHAIKH *et al.*, 2002).

Wounds are injuries resulting from aggression against soft tissues, caused by traumatic agents that damage them. In general, wounds cause pain, bleeding of varying intensities and the risk of infection. These injuries can be classified according to the etiological factor, degree of contamination, type of healing, complexity, degree of opening, time of evolution, tissue involvement and mechanism of injury (CLARK *et al.*, 1996).

Soft tissue injuries can be classified into: (1) abrasion or abrasion, which is a superficial injury to the skin characterized by the loss of the epithelium and exposure of the connective tissue (TAHER *et al.*, 1998); (2) cutting wounds, which are those that result from sharp objects (knives, razors and blades) sliding over the tissues (LEITE SEGUNDO *et al., 2007); (3) puncture wounds, which are caused by* sharp objects with a uniform diameter, such as nails, needles and ice picks (ZAVA *et al., 2010),* 2007); (3) puncture wounds, which are caused by sharp objects with a uniform diameter, such as nails, needles and ice picks (ZAVA *et al.,* 2010); (4) avulsive wounds, which are produced when the agent causing the trauma causes a rupture with partial or total loss of tissue continuity in the anatomical region (QUIRINO *et al., 2010); (5)* avulsive wounds, which are produced when the agent causing the trauma causes a rupture with partial or total loss of tissue continuity in the anatomical region (QUIRINO *et al., 2010),* 2010); (5) blunt wounds, which have irregular, sinuous and star-shaped margins, as they are produced by blunt objects, by means of compression, traction, percussion and dragging forces (CHAIA *et al.*, 2013); (6) puncture-cut wounds, which are conditions caused by a mixed action mechanism, with a linear aspect and a slit-like shape, such as knives and daggers (DANTAS *et al.,* 2013); (7) puncture-contact wounds, which are those with a piercing and blunt action mechanism at the same time (QUIRINO *et al., 2010),* 2010); (8) cut-contusion wounds, which have an action mechanism that is both sharp and blunt at the same time, such as a scythe, machete and axe (NOGUEIRA *et al.,* 2015); and finally (9) lacero-contusion wounds, which are most often caused by compression action mechanisms, i.e. the crushing of the skin and associated tissue loss (ZAVA *et al.,* 2010).

In view of the above, the aim of this study was to evaluate the clinical and epidemiological profile and characteristics of soft tissue injuries in patients who were victims of oral and maxillofacial (BMF) trauma in a Brazilian population.

Mortality due to traffic accidents and transportation in Pernambuco

Traffic accidents have a huge impact on the health of the population and have a direct impact on the quality of life and life expectancy of adolescents, young people and adults. As a result, they entail high social costs in terms of health treatment, especially curative and rehabilitative procedures, as well as taking individuals away from their work, studies and social life (WHO, 2007).

Brazil ranks 5th[a] among the nations with a high mortality rate related to traffic and transport accidents. Pernambuco ranks 10th in the number of victims of motorcycle accidents, with a rate of 9.6 per 100,000 inhabitants (BRASIL, MS, 2013).

The Pernambuco State Health Department (SES) recorded 45,916 traffic accidents, 75% of which were fatal. According to the state's traffic department (DETRAN), speeding is the most common offense, followed by running red lights (SES-PE, 2013).

According to the bulletin on land transport accidents from January to November 2013, the IX Health Region, to which the municipality of Trindade belongs, ranked first in the state of Pernambuco, by health region, with an accident rate of 79.7 per 10,000 inhabitants. The municipality of Trindade has a rate of 50.4 and is among the highest in this region. In 2012, the regional committee for the prevention of motorcycle accidents (CRPAM) was set up in this health region, comprising the Regional Health Management, Military Police, Fire Brigade, Federal Highway Police, Regional DETRAN and IBAMA (SES-PE, 2013).

The cost of traffic accidents in Pernambuco; 650 million were spent on injuries and deaths from traffic accidents in Pernambuco in 2012, 2013 and 2014, there was a 13% increase in motorcycle accidents alone in 2014, 46,000 injuries were treated by the state (not all are hospitalized) 34,000 injuries were victims of motorcycle accidents for every 4 people injured in traffic, 3 were on a motorcycle (DIARIO DE PERNAMBUCO, 2014).

Oral and Maxillofacial Injuries caused by Interpersonal Violence.

Accidental and intentional trauma, especially physical aggression, are major problems in today's society. Records from the World Health Organization indicate that trauma is among the main causes of morbidity and mortality, affecting the population with great epidemiological variability, regardless of age, gender, income or geographical location. Facial injuries represent a significant injury to health worldwide, with a high incidence and diversity in form and severity (OLIVEIRA *et al.,* 2008).

Violence is considered to exist when there is a situation of interaction in which one or more actors act directly or indirectly. Currently, crime rates are increasingly high and generate intense debate in various sectors of society and concomitantly contribute to raising the mortality rate. The number of homicides in Brazil increased considerably between 1991 and 2000, by around 50% according to the Ministry of Health's mortality information system (SIM) (MINISTERIO DA SAUDE, 2005).

In 2013, the municipality of Trindade had 26 cases of death caused by violence, making it the highest homicide rate among those that make up the IX Regional Health Management (IX GERES) (SES-PE, 2013).

The craniofacial integument and osseous framework, due to their anterior projection in relation to the body, are extremely exposed to aggression from violence and other causes. The soft tissues of the face are compressed between the bones and external aggression forces, and are forced to break, generating countless injuries (cuts, lacerations, hemorrhages, hematomas, etc.), which can vary in shape, extent, depth and severity (VIEIRA *et al.,* 2013).

CHAPTER 2

General Aspects of Injuries to the Maxillofacial Complex

Injuries to the soft tissues of the face are frequently encountered in the care of polytraumatized patients. Injuries can be restricted to the superficial layers of the skin or extend to muscles, bones, vessels, nerves, salivary glands and alveolar-dental structures. These injuries can be classified as abrasions, contusions, avulsions, incisions, lacerations, punctures, bites and burns (FONSECA et al., 2015).

In the care of these patients, airway maintenance, control of bleeding and stabilization of injuries to other important systems should be prioritized before assessing facial injuries (HUPP *et al.,* 2015).

Given the large vascularization of the head and neck region, injuries tend to generate bleeding, however, given the smaller caliber of the vessels, this tends to stop spontaneously, persistent bleeding responds well to local hemostatic maneuvers, such as compression, vessel ligation and electrocoagulation (FONSECA et al., 2015).

Wounds can also be classified as clean or contaminated. However, clean wounds can become contaminated as the time of exposure after trauma increases, and late approaches also favor contamination. Contaminated wounds require antibiotic therapy. Contamination usually occurs with strains of *Streptococcus* and *Staphylococcus,* when there is a solution of continuity and communication of the wound with the intra-oral and extra-oral environment (PRADO *et al.,* 2004).

Anti-tetanus immunization should also be administered to contaminated lesions. Patients with adequate vaccination coverage, a full course of 03 doses of Diphtheria and Tetanus (DT) vaccine within a 10-year period do not need a booster dose (0.5 ml) intramuscularly (IM). For those with no history of immunization, they should undergo the full course (03 doses), those who have completed the full course and are more than 10 years from the last dose should receive the booster dose and those who even less than 10 years from the last dose have extensive wounds, with the presence of a foreign body or exposed to contaminated materials, should also receive the booster dose. Major injuries and contamination should be assessed for the need to administer Antitetanus Serum 5000 IU, IM (SAT) (FONSECA et al., 2015).

The injuries with the highest risk of developing Tetanus are those with more than 6 hours of exposure, depth greater than 1 cm, firearm injuries (FAF), stab wounds (FAB), burns, crushing, necrotic, exudative and with the presence of contaminants (dust, feces, soil and saliva) (HUPP et al., 2015).

The management of these lesions includes copious washing with saline solution, removal of foreign bodies and dirt. Wounds with necrotic edges should be debrided before final treatment, and the beard and scalp region should be trichotomized for better assessment and reference during repositioning (FONSECA et al., 2015).

2.1 Etiology of Oral and Maxillofacial Injuries

Traumatic injuries to the soft tissues of the maxillofacial region are higher than injuries to other regions of the body, due to the exposure of its structures and the lack of protection. The causes of trauma to the face vary and can be related to factors such as age, gender, social status and geographical location, among others. Traffic and transportation accidents (TTAs), interpersonal violence, falls, sports practice and accidents at work are the main causes. The treatment of facial injuries is aimed at restoring function and minimizing the consequences for the patient's appearance (RODRIGUES *et al.,* 2006).

In the care of polytraumatized patients and other emergency situations, cranio-maxillofacial injuries are a very important circumstance in the care provided, since their severity can compromise human life. This is coupled with the fact that when poorly managed, injuries leave both aesthetic and functional sequelae and can isolate the individual from their social relationships (VIEIRA *et al.,* 2013).

Facial trauma is a common clinical situation in emergency units and hospitals, especially in large urban centers and in regions with increased demand for mobility, associated with traffic violations and growing levels of crime (MARZOLA *et al.,* 2008).

Facial wounds come in many forms and vary in complexity, depending on their extent, depth, degree of contamination, etiologic agent and exposure time. These wounds should be treated as quickly as possible. The risk of infection and unsatisfactory aesthetics are related to injuries with longer tissue exposure times (JARDIM *et al.,* 2010).

2.2 Classification of Soft Tissue Injuries.

Wounds are injuries resulting from aggression against soft tissues, caused by traumatic agents that damage them. In general, wounds cause pain, bleeding of varying intensities and the risk of infection. They can be classified according to the etiological factor, degree of contamination, type of healing, complexity, degree of opening, time of evolution, tissue involvement and mechanism of injury (CHAIA *et al.,* 2013).

Injuries can originate from four categories of traumatic agents: mechanical (restraint, puncture, cut, etc.); physical (cold, heat and radiation); chemical (chemical products) and mixed (FONSECA *et al.*, 2015).

2.2.1 Classification of facial injuries according to the mechanism of injury.

Table 1. Classification of injuries according to mechanism of action

ISOLATED LESIONS	*ASSOCIATED INJURIES*
ABRASION/SCORING	SHARPS
INCISED OR SHARP	PUNCTURE WOUNDS
PIERCING OR PENETRATING	CORTO CONTUSA
AVULSIVE	LACERO CONTUSA
CONTUSA	

Abrasion or abrasion is a superficial skin lesion characterized by the loss of the epidermis due to trauma, resulting from sudden contact with a rough surface, an ill-defined margin, and usually a foreign body in the lesion. It is extremely painful due to the exposure of the conjunctival layer and nerve fibers, but the prognosis is favorable (HUPP *et al.*, 2015).

Sharp wounds are those that result from sharp objects (knives, razors and blades) sliding across the tissue. They are usually deep with uniform edges and with length predominating over depth (FONSECA *et al.*, 2015).

Puncture wounds are caused by sharp objects with a uniform diameter, such as nails, needles and ice picks. These wounds present as a bleeding point, without major tissue damage, but in depth they can reach vital organs (PRADO *et al.,* 2004).

The avulsive wound is produced when the agent causing the trauma causes partial or total laceration of the anatomical region. **Blunt wounds** have irregular, sinuous and star-shaped margins, as they are produced by blunt objects, by means of compression, traction, percussion and dragging (CHAIA *et al.,* 2013).

Sharps injuries are injuries caused by a mixed action mechanism, with a linear appearance and a slit shape. They are usually caused by objects such as knives and daggers. **Puncture-contact wounds** are those with both a piercing and blunt mechanism of action. It has a more or less blunt edge, or soon takes on this character. This injury is typical of gunshot wounds, which perforate due to the force that hits the skin surface and are blunt due to their shape. The aspects of this injury vary depending on the caliber of the gun and the distance from which it was fired (FONSECA *etal.,* 2015).

Cut-contusion wounds have an action mechanism that is both sharp and blunt, like a scythe, machete or axe. **Lacero-contusous wounds** are most often caused by compression action mechanisms, i.e. the skin crushing against the underlying plane, or penetration by tearing or lacerating the tissue, with irregular edges at more than one angle, an example of which is a dog bite (HUPP *et al.,* 2015).

2.3-Treatment

Before establishing clinical-surgical therapy for facial injuries, the patient should be assessed to rule out the presence of life-threatening injuries. The patient should be fully approached and the situation should be checked beyond soft tissue injuries, after which priorities should be established and actions planned with a view to the best time for intervention, ruling out possible facial fractures and/or other conditions that could lead to complications, such as anti-tetanus immunization (CHAIA *et al.,* 2013).

2.3.1-Cleaning the wound

Thorough cleaning of the wound is of fundamental importance in order to achieve good healing and minimize the risk of infection. The wound should be flushed with 0.9% saline solution to remove clots, foreign bodies and exogenous material. Antiseptic solutions such as polyvinyl-pyrrolidone-iodine (PVPI) and hydrogen peroxide ($H2O2$) should not be used because they are caustic and cytotoxic and cause tissue damage, but they may be indicated for infected wounds and abscesses (VALLDERRAMA *et al.,* 2006).

2.3.2 Hemostasis

Hemostasis is a set of maneuvers designed to stop or prevent bleeding. Hemostasis must be effective in preventing the formation of hematomas and dead spaces. Compression maneuvers with surgical gauze or compresses over the wound area promote temporary hemostasis. Maintaining compression for five minutes facilitates definitive hemostasis, which can be achieved by occluding the vessels with delicate hemostatic drops (Kelly, Halsted, Crile, Mixter and Rochester) and then suturing the vessel, achieving definitive hemostasis (SANTOS *et al.,* 2011).

2.3.3 Debridement

It involves removing unviable (necrotic) tissue and smoothing the edges of the wound, reducing the risk of infection and the possibility of deforming scars, respectively. Resections of macerated or necrotic tissues should be carried out with a very sharp scalpel or scissors, preserving wet tissue, in order to favor the repair of the injury. The presence of necrotic tissue increases the risk of infection and masks the extent and depth of the wound (DANTAS *et al.,* 2013).

2.3.4-Suture

The tissues must be slit using delicate and suitable material. The edges of the tissues must be joined by anatomical planes, in order to prevent the formation of dead space. This minimizes the formation of tension forces and properly restores and repositions the layers, which favors the regeneration of the affected nerve fibers. The approximation of the deep planes (muscular and subcutaneous) is essential to facilitate the return to function of the muscles of facial expression, which are important in aesthetic-functional repair (LEITE SEGUNDO *et al.,* 2007).

For facial sutures, threads should be used that provide good approximation of the wound edges, smaller marks on the skin and less foreign body reaction, as well as the least traumatic needles possible. The suture thread should preferably cause minimal irritation to the tissues, causing a low-intensity, short-lived inflammatory response. The threads indicated for the treatment of facial wounds are polyglactin 910 (Vicryl®/Ethicon - Johnson & Johnson and Monocryl®/Ethicon - Johnson & Johnson) and nylon (Mononylon®/Ethicon - Johnson & Johnson) (DANTAS *et al.,* 2013).

2.3.5 Use of Antibiotics

The use of antibiotics in surgical interventions can be prophylactic or therapeutic, with the aim of preventing and treating surgical wound infection. The maintenance of antibiotic therapy is necessary in the management of contaminated or potentially contaminated wounds. Wounds that do not require antibiotic therapy should be instructed on how to clean the wound. In contaminated wounds located in the oral region, the use of antibiotics is indicated selectively, according to the condition of the wound, type of exposure, as well as the patient's systemic condition (CHAIA *et al.,* 2013).

The efficacy of antibiotics in cases of open wounds is questionable, because the drug only comes into contact with the tissues after contamination, which is important for establishing the duration of treatment, linked to factors in the body such as a decrease in defense capacity linked to systemic and local conditions (PRADO *et al.,* 2004).

Generally, the antibiotics used are betalactams, Amoxicillin and Ampicillin (penicillins) and Cephalexin and Ceftriaxone (Cephalosporins). The former are more suitable for lesions in the oral cavity. The use of cephalosporins, especially ceftriaxone, is indicated for intravenous (IV) therapy for patients with facial wounds in a hospital environment, while cephalexin can be administered orally (VO) to patients who have been discharged from hospital (BUCHER *et al.,* 2011).

In patients allergic to penicillins, the antibiotic of choice is Clindamycin, a drug from the lincosamide class, which has good penetration in bone tissue and broad coverage against gran negative microorganisms. Another option is Azithromycin, which belongs to the azalide class (CHAIA *et al.,* 2013).

Table 2. Antibiotic therapy regimens

AMOXICILLIN 500mg orally (VO)	8/8 hours for 7 days
AMPICILLIN 500mg intravenous (IV)	6/6 hours for 5 days
CEFALEXIN 500 mg VO	6/6 hours for 7 days
CEFALOTIN 1g IV	6/6 hours for 3-5 days
CEFTRIAXONE 1g IV	12/12 hours for 3-5 days

CLINDAMICIN 300 mg VO	8/8 hours for 07 days
CLINDAMICIN 600 mg/ml	8/8 hours for 3 - 5 days
AZITHROMYCIN 500mg	24/24 hours 3-5 days

2.3.6- Immunization

When caring for patients with facial injuries, the patient's immunization status should be assessed. As these injuries present a potential risk of contamination, caused by accidents that can carry dendrites to exposed tissues, anti-tetanus immunoprophylaxis should always be instituted. Tetanus is caused by *Clostridium tetani,* a gram-positive bacillus commonly found in soil and animal waste. Factors such as the degree of contamination of the wound and the individual's vaccination status should be considered. The prophylactic regimen should be indicated for non-immunized patients, especially when they have lacerocontusion wounds, transfixion wounds and firearm puncture wounds (PRADO *et al.,* 2004).

2.4 - Assisting patients with facial injuries and facial trauma

Although soft tissue injuries of the face are not commonly associated with a risk of death, they play an important role in the care of polytraumatized patients, because when they are poorly repaired, they remove the individual from the social bed, marginalizing them (VIEIRA *et al.,* 2013).

Facial trauma is an urgent and emergency situation present in emergency units and hospitals all over the world, especially in places with high rates of violence and traffic offenses. In this broad area of care, facial trauma includes soft tissue and associated bones, with or without the retention of foreign bodies (MARZOLA *et al.,* 2008).

The principles of care are based on the severity of the trauma and, based on this, a sequence of procedures is established, in stages, which can be carried out concurrently. One of the instruments used to assess the degree of impairment and general condition of the patient is the Glasgow coma scale, which, depending on the score for the clinical situation, directs the intervention measures applied to the patient, with the aim of identifying the severity of their clinical situation through the patient's responses (CARRASCO *et al.,* 2012).

Facial trauma is closely related to polytrauma and the repair of soft tissue injuries is addressed after the patient has been stabilized. Clinical-surgical therapy of injuries is a priority when they are related to noble structures and offer potential risk to the patient in the face of complications to systemic health, such as in cases of severe bleeding and injuries associated with upper airway patency, thus assuming the need for immediate intervention (MARZOLA *et al.,* 2008).

2.5-Injuries Associated with Dento-Alveolar Trauma

Trauma can be conceptualized as an interruption in tissue continuity, and healing is the process of re-establishing this continuity. The result can be either tissue repair, in which continuity is restored, but the scar tissue is anatomically and functionally distinct, or tissue regeneration, in which both anatomy and function are restored (MELO *et al.,* 2003).

Dento-alveolar trauma has a significant incidence among the traumas that affect the face. They can be classified according to a wide variety of factors, such as: etiology, anatomy, pathology, therapy, among others. These injuries affect the teeth, pulp, periodontal tissues, alveolar bone and oral mucosa (MELO *et al.,*

2003).

Dental traumas are urgent dental incidents that require the professional to provide quick but thorough care. Despite the promptness of the first treatment, in most cases the patient needs to be followed up for a long period of time. The incidence of this type of injury ranges from 4 to 30% in the general population. Dental injuries can be associated with bone fractures, injuries to the soft tissues of the face and other facial injuries (VASCONCELLOS *et al.,* 2006).

When facial injuries are associated with dento-alveolar trauma, it is essential to check that there is no foreign body lodged in the adjacent soft tissue. This is particularly evident in cases where the patient has bitten the soft tissue and where tooth fractures are evident; enamel fragments may be embedded in the soft tissue (DYM *et al.,* 2004).

According to Andreasen and Andreasen (2001), dento-alveolar trauma can be classified into a system that includes the tooth, periodontal tissue, gums and oral mucosa and damage to the supporting bone. This classification was recommended because it is easy to memorize and the dental trauma is logically ordered as follows: CORONARY FRACTURES: Enamel crack, enamel fracture, enamel and dentin fracture and enamel, dentin and pulp fracture. CORONO-RADICULAR FRACTURES: Uncomplicated crown and root fracture and complicated crown and root fracture. RADICULAR FRACTURES: Horizontal and oblique fractures, cervical tergus, middle tergus, apical tergus and vertical fractures. INJURIES INVOLVING TEETH AND SUPPORTING PERIODONTAL TISSUES: Concussion, subluxation, lateral luxation, extrusive luxation, intrusion and avulsion.

2.6- **Firearm injuries**

With the increase in crime rates, firearm puncture wounds (FAP) are increasingly common in the urgent and emergency sectors of hospital units. These injuries require a multidisciplinary approach due to their complexity and the imminent risk of death for patients. When they hit the craniofacial region, they have serious repercussions due to the risk of damage to noble structures, impairment of the upper airways and damage to the encephalon (SOUZA JUNIOR *et al.*, 2018).

Brazil occupies second place in firearm-related deaths in a ranking of 52 countries listed by UNESCO. Brazilian rates are so high that they exceed those seen in war zones such as those in Africa and the Middle East (SANCHES *et al.*, 2009). Within the context of trauma care, firearm injuries are the second leading cause of death, surpassed only by traffic accidents (PEREIRA *et al.*, 2006).

Facial injuries caused by firearms result in significant damage to the tissues of the oral and maxillofacial complex and constitute a challenge in their approach and repair, being responsible for high morbidity and mortality, as they compromise the patient's life, function and aesthetics. Firearm-related puncture wounds can be classified as perforated-contusions, as they are shaped by the action of blunt-ended agents, which perforate through the force of impact due to their displacement and contusion at the same time (LEITE SEGUNDO *et al.*, 2013).

These injuries are extremely variable in pattern, causing serious damage to vital structures, significant bleeding and impairment of respiratory and neurological functions. Damage to the architecture of the soft tissues of the face generally occurs with loss of substance, irregularity of the edges and transfixation of the planes, and can present exit holes or become lodged in the face or skull (PEREIRA *et al.*, 2006).

When dealing with firearm injuries to the maxillofacial complex, the initial maneuvers should be aimed at maintaining the airways, which may be compromised by obstruction or direct damage, and at controlling any bleeding present. Once the patient's condition has stabilized, imaging tests should be carried out to assess the size of the injuries and the wounds should be managed with copious cleaning to remove necrotic tissue and fragments of projectiles, which are sources of infection (PEREIRA *et al.*, 2006).

Correction of fractures and other injuries should be instituted as soon as the patient's clinical condition is stable, antibiotic therapy should be employed and antitetanus chemoprophylaxis is of paramount importance given the risk that these injuries present for the development of Tetanus (SOUZA JUNIOR *et al.*, 2018).

2.7- White Weapon Wounds

Interpersonal violence is a serious public health problem in Brazil and around the world, due to its repercussions on sectors of society such as public security, and in this context we can mention stab wounds.Since the maxillofacial region is often affected by traumatic injuries associated or not with bodily injuries, injuries resulting from the actions of knife blades are uncommon, given voluntary self-protection actions, where the individual protects the face with the use of the upper limbs (NOGUEIRA NETO JN *et al.*, 2015).

Stab wounds penetrate different anatomical structures and the removal of the artifacts that cause them, when lodged, is judicious and potentially fatal, especially with regard to vascular injuries. The approach to these situations must be multidisciplinary, starting with maintaining airway patency, hemodynamic stabilization, and neurological and ophthalmic assessment if necessary, and this conduct is associated with the need for imaging tests to assess the location of the object and affected structures (ZANDOMENIGHI *et al.*, 2014).

2.8 - Burns to the Maxillofacial Complex

Burns can be defined as injuries caused by thermal, chemical, electrical or radioactive agents that affect the body's lining tissues, compromising tissue integrity and reaching deeper structures such as fat, muscle and bone tissue. These injuries are extremely painful, generating physical and psychological sequelae (BARRETO *et al.*, 2011).

First-degree burns are those that affect the epidermis, with erythema, edema and mild to moderate pain as clinical manifestations. Second-degree lesions affect the epidermis and dermis, along with the vasculo-nervous structures in this layer. These have devitalized tissue, bleeding and intense pain, and blistering is common (TELES et al., 2012). Third-degree lesions reach the deepest layers, compromising all layers of the lining tissue, reaching muscle tissue and exposing bone (ALCANTARA *et al.*, 2009).

Burns involving the face and neck are considered to be critical injuries, and are highly serious due to the high risk of infection and the potential sequelae generated, which require immediate and specific treatment. The face is considered a critical region because it contains noble structures such as eyeballs, nose, mouth and ears, and has rich innervation and vascularization (DORNELAS, FERREIRA E CAZARIM, 2009).

Patients who are victims of burns to the face require rigorous assessment. In the case of second and third degree burns, the patient must be kept under observation in a hospital environment and, depending on the severity of the case, remain hospitalized for damage assessment, antibiotic coverage and minimization of sequelae. The first few hours are of great importance because the edema generated can compromise the upper airways, causing respiratory failure (DORNELAS, FERREIRA E CAZARIM, 2009).

The first care provided is copious irrigation of the lesions with 0.9% saline solution, removal of devitalized tissue if possible at the time, trichotomy if necessary, elevated headboard 30-45 degrees, maintenance of airway patency and oxygen therapy via nasal catheter or Venturi mask. In extensive, second or third degree burns, venous hydration should be instituted, along with broad-spectrum antibiotic therapy (BOLGIANI E SERRA, 2010).

The wound bed should be treated with topical agents, such as 1% silver sulphadiazine ointment or collagenase, both of which have antibiotic action and act as a chemical debridement, stimulating healing. For best results, dressings should be changed twice a day. More superficial lesions tend to heal in up to two weeks, while deeper lesions may require reconstructive procedures such as skin grafts (BOLGIANI E SERRA, 2010).

The risk of infection and damage to the noble structures of the face are complications that can occur, making therapy and rehabilitation more complex and requiring a specialized professional approach. The main consequences of facial burns are scar retraction, which can lead to microstomia, interfering with the functions of the stomatognathic system, such as swallowing, phonation and facial expression, as well as paresthesia, dysesthesia or paralysis (ALCANTARA *et al.,* 2009).

2.9 - Bites to the face

Injuries caused by bites are the most common injuries seen in hospital emergency departments, accounting for around 1% of cases. However, only 10% of victims require specialized treatment or hospitalization (MACEDO E SILVA, 2018).

Bites can be caused by animals and humans. These wounds can be irregular in shape when there is a mechanism for bringing tissue in during the bite, or they can have the shape of the attacker's teeth and dental arch (MACEDO

E SILVA, 2018).

The main complication linked to these injuries is contamination and, if they are caused by animals that are hosts of the human rabies virus, a zoonosis transmitted to humans by some species of domestic animals, such as dogs and cats, wild animals such as monkeys and bats, and production animals such as horses and cattle (MACEDO E SILVA, 2018).

Rabies is a serious infectious disease caused by a virus of the *Lyssavirus* genus, of the *Rhabdoviridae* family, which leads to the death of almost 100% of infected patients. Rabies is a zoonosis, also known as hydrophobia, where the virus is transmitted through the saliva of infected animals. Bites to the head or neck are much more serious because they are close to the brain (MIRANDA E MOREIRA, 2003).

There is no cure for human rabies. In cases of exposure to the virus through animal bites, chemoprophylaxis with rabies vaccine should be used. The schedule follows a protocol of 5 doses to be administered at an interval of 28 days (0, 3, 7, 14 and 28), and in the most serious cases, the administration of anti-rabies serum (SAR) should be indicated (MIRANDA E MOREIRA, 2003).

CHAPTER 3.

RESEARCH METHODOLOGY

This study is relevant given the need to identify the main etiologies of facial trauma, and since this is a multifactorial complex, preventive and executable strategies must be formulated in order to protect and rehabilitate human health. The survey of data on the subject provides information on the circumstances and agents involved, pointing out the main complications presented by the victims, thus exposing clinical situations that require specialized assistance. The context addresses the main causes of facial injuries, which are traffic accidents, interpersonal violence and domestic accidents (falls), and thus becomes a source of reference for future studies on the subject and a basis for the formulation of prevention and health promotion actions.

OBJECTIVES

General Objective

- To evaluate the prevalence and characteristics of soft tissue injuries in the cranio-maxillofacial region in a public hospital.

Specific Objectives

- 1-Perform an epidemiological analysis of the causes of craniofacial injuries.
    - 2-Evaluate the clinical approach to patients with traumatic facial injuries.
    - 3-Evaluate the treatment techniques applied to injuries.
- 4-Gather data that can be used to formulate and implement public policies aimed at preventing accidents and interpersonal violence.

METHODOLOGY

Research location

The Maria Veneri Municipal Hospital, located in Trindade - PE, is a small health unit belonging to the municipal health department (SMS), which provides urgent and emergency care for adults and children, as well as medical, pediatric and obstetric care. The clinical staff is made up of nursing professionals and on-call doctors. The unit provides low-complexity care and is a reference for the municipality's family health units. When medium and high-complexity care is required, users are referred to the Fernando Bezerra Regional Hospital in Ouricuri, which is a state hospital. The HMMV provides an average of 150 visits a day and is part of the IX Regional Health Management of the state of Pernambuco (GERES).

Sample

The convenience sample consisted of patients treated in the urgent and emergency department of the HMMV from June 2014 to June 2015, totaling 213 cases, distributed by gender in the following age groups: 0 to 12, 12 to 18, 18 to 30, 30 to 55 and 55 years or older.

Inclusion and Exclusion Criteria

Inclusion criteria: records of patients who had been seen in the urgent and emergency department of the HMMV and had suffered an injury to the maxillofacial region between 06/2014 and 06/2015.

Exclusion criteria: medical records with incomplete information on the trauma suffered by patients seen in the department who had not suffered injuries to the maxillofacial region.

Ethical aspects of research

In order to carry out this study, it was assessed and approved by the Research Ethics Committee of the Centro Universitario Doutor Leao Sampaio - CEP/UNILEAO (protocol no. 1.429.294).

Data collection

The information was collected from the medical records and shift reports of the department and recorded on a maxillofacial trauma assessment form developed by the researchers and distributed according to the causative agent and the nature of the trauma, the type, location and extent of the injury, based on figure 1, as well as the treatment applied and the fate of the patient.

Figure 01: Anatomical division of the face: (1) frontal region; (2) parietal region; (3) occipital region; (4) temporal region; (5) orbital region; (6) nasal region; (7) infraorbital region; (8) zygomatic region; (9) parotidomastoid region; (10) cheek region; (11) buccal region; (12) mentual region.

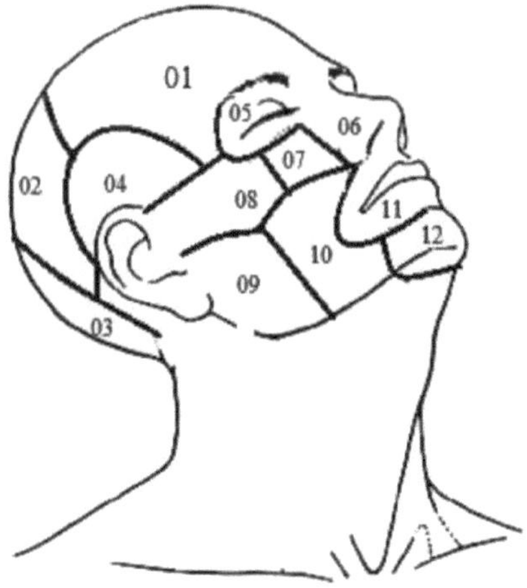

Data Analysis

Descriptive statistics were used, the data was computerized and tabulated in spreadsheets using the Office Excel 2010 program, the statistical calculations were carried out using SPSS software version 17.0, evaluating the quantitative data in terms of mean and percentage for each variable and formulating tables and graphs.

Medical records of patients with a history of oral and maxillofacial trauma between June 2014 and June 2015 were included in the study. Incomplete or illegible records were excluded from the study. The work team consisted of two previously trained undergraduate dental students (S.E.S.M and M.I.L). The data obtained was entered and tabulated in the SPSS program version 17.0 *(Statistical Package for Social Science)* and then treated with descriptive statistical tests.

CHAPTER 4.

RESULTS

Of the 213 cases selected for the study, 173 (81.2%) were male and 40 (18.8%) female, with an average age of 29.8 years (median 27 years), ranging from 02 to 76 years old.

With regard to the etiological factor of oral and maxillofacial trauma, motorcycle accidents were the most prevalent cause of facial soft tissue injuries, accounting for 46.9% (n=100) of the sample, followed by physical assaults (20.7%, n=44) and falls (10.3%, n=22). In addition, cases of cycling accidents, pedestrian accidents, car accidents and stab wounds were also identified (Table 01).

TABLE 1: Distribution of the sample according to the etiological agents of oral and maxillofacial trauma.

CAUSE OF TRAUMA	N	PERCENTAGE
Motorcycle accident	100	46,9%
Physical aggression	44	20,7%
Fall	22	10,3%
Cycling accident	12	5,6%
Hit-and-run	09	4,2
Car accident	08	3,8%
Gunshot wound white	04	1,9%
Other*	14	6,6%

Sports accidents, animal accidents, construction accidents

Of the patients who had an injury to the face, taking the topography of the soft tissue injuries as a reference, the most commonly affected areas were the frontal region (20.7%, n=44) followed by the cheek region (16%, n=34) and the orbital region (15.5%, n=33). Lesions were also found in the occipital, parietal, buccal, zygomatic, temporal and nasal regions (Table 02).

TAB. 2: Distribution of the sample according to the site of the oral and maxillofacial trauma.

ANATOMICAL SITE	N	PERCENTAL
Front	44	20,7%
Cheek	34	16%
Orbital	33	15,5%
Occipital	23	10,8%
Parietal	19	8,9%
Mouth	16	7,5%
Zygomatics	16	7,5%
Mentual	14	6,6%
Temporal	08	3,8%
Nasal	06	2,8%

Analysis of the type of injury caused by the trauma showed that the most prevalent injuries were blunt injuries, which were identified in 91 patients (42.7%). Excoriations were the second most common type of injury in the sample, accounting for 16.9% (n=36), followed by cut and laceration injuries (11.3%, n=24) (Table 03).

TAB. 3: Distribution of the sample according to the type of injury caused by the oral and maxillofacial trauma.

TYPE OF INJURY	N	PERCENTAGE
Corto-contusa	91	42,7%
Slagging/abrasion	36	16,9%
Cutting	24	11,3%
Lacero-contusa	24	11,3%
Hematoma	21	9,9%
Sharps	10	4,7%
Puncture wounds	7	3,3%

The treatment of choice for the majority of cases was suturing and dressings (77.5%, n=165). For 85.4% of the patients (n=182) the trauma progressed to hospital discharge. Transfer of the victim to highly complex hospitals occurred in 14.6% of the sample (n=31). With regard to dental involvement, only 2.8% of the cases studied had any trauma to the dental organ.

CHAPTER 5.

DISCUSSION

In the care of polytraumatized patients, oral and maxillofacial injuries are relevant to the care of the victim, since the severity of the injuries can put human life at risk (CARVALHO *et al.,* 2010). The literature emphasizes that the initial clinical approach in the care of individuals with trauma to the maxillofacial complex should focus on a thorough clinical examination in order to rule out the presence of life-threatening injuries PETERSON, (2004). In many situations, imaging tests such as X-rays, CT scans and ultrasounds are necessary to better assess the patient's clinical condition (CHAIA *et al.,* 2013).

The results of the study showed that oral and maxillofacial injuries were more prevalent in males and that the most common cause of trauma was motorcycle accidents. In Brazil, men make up the majority of the population who drive vehicles, especially motorcycles (CHAIA *et al.,* 2013). In this sense, males are more likely to be involved in traffic accidents. In addition, the lack of use of protective equipment such as helmets and seat belts, as well as the consumption of alcoholic beverages may contribute to the high prevalence of trauma involving injuries to the soft tissues of the oral and maxillofacial complex in this group of people (ROSELINO *et al.,* 2009).

The anatomical location and type of trauma are important predictors of injury severity (ZAVA *et al.,* 2010; CHAIA *et al.,* 2013). In the present study, the most commonly affected anatomical sites were the frontal, orbital and cheek regions. The literature describes that the location and prevalence of injuries in the oral-facial region may be related to skeletal projections of the skull and face (VIEIRA *et al.,* 2013). This factor is linked to the fact that in trauma resulting from accidents involving vehicles, the biomechanics involved at the time of the frontal and/or lateral impact more often expose the middle and upper tergium of the face (PETERSON, 2004). As for the type of injury caused by the trauma, it was observed that blunt injuries were the most prevalent. Several authors have stated that the type of injury caused by trauma depends on the type and strength of the causative agent (ZAVA *et al.,* 2010; CHAIA *et al.,* 2013). Injuries to soft tissue occur primarily through compression of the tissue between the bones and the blunt object and, depending on the incidence of the force and the shape of the object, the most diverse forms of injury occur (VIEIRA *et al,* 2013).

Several authors emphasize that the management of oral and facial wounds should be guided by the principles of hemorrhage containment (compression, ligation of vessels) as well as infection prevention (LEITE SEGUNDO *et al.,* 2007; JARDIN et al., 2010; QUIRINO et *al.,* 2010). Cleaning wounds is of fundamental importance for minimizing the risk of infection. Many studies state that wounds should be washed with 0.9% saline solution in order to remove clots, foreign bodies and exogenous materials (VALDERRAMA *et al.,* 2006; SANTOS *et al.,* 2011; SHAIKH et *al.,* 2002). Several authors point out that the longer the wound is exposed, the greater the potential for infection (ZAVA et *al.,* 2010; QUIRINO *et a.l,* 2010; CHAIA *et al.,* 2013). In addition, injuries associated with macerations and/or ischemia may present an increased risk of infection (BOLT *et al.,* 2004). The presence of necrotic tissue also increases the risk of infection and masks the extent and depth of the wound (DANTAS *et al.,* 2013).

In this study, the procedure of choice for most patients was suturing followed by hospital discharge. These findings suggest that an immediate approach with dressings and sutures and infection control maneuvers are generally effective in cases of soft tissue injuries to the mouth and face. The literature emphasizes that when suturing tissues, threads should be used that provide good approximation to the edges of the wound, low potential for scar formation and minimal irritation to the tissues (LEITE SEGUNDO *et al.,* 2007; PETERSON, 2004; ZAVA et *al.,* 2010; CHAIA *et al.,* 2013; SINGER et *al.,* 2005).

Interestingly, only 2.8% of the sample had any associated dental trauma. Some studies indicate that dento-alveolar trauma can have an incidence of between 4 and 30% in the general population (PETERSON, 2004; MELO *et al.,* 2003). This data may differ from the literature due to the following factors: the hospital unit in which this study was carried out does not have a dental professional for trauma care; and the professional usually responsible for this care is a medical professional, a general practitioner who does not specialize in maxillofacial trauma and intraoral examination is not routine in his daily practice.

Due to the high prevalence and incidence of facial trauma, it is necessary to have a broad understanding of the patterns of injuries that affect the face, so that emergency care is as effective as possible, in order to provide appropriate conduct and treatment (BOLT *et al.*, 2004).

Injuries to the soft tissues of the face are a clinical situation of great importance in patients who are victims of oral and maxillofacial trauma, due to their complexity, since injuries of this type can generate aesthetic and functional sequelae. This requires an affective approach and a great deal of knowledge on the part of the emergency professional, whether a doctor or an oral and maxillofacial surgeon (CHAIA *et al.,* 2013).

This study is relevant because there are still few clinical-epidemiological studies on soft tissue injuries caused by trauma to the maxillofacial complex. It could form the basis for future research, as well as elucidating important concepts regarding the care of patients who are victims of these injuries.

CHAPTER 6.

CONCLUSION

Based on the data presented in this study, we can conclude that: men are involved in traffic accidents and interpersonal violence more often than women, especially young adults. Motorcycle accidents are the most common cause (46.9%) of facial trauma, followed by physical aggression (20.7%) and falls from height (10.3%). The most prevalent injury is the blunt type (42.7%).

The most commonly affected anatomical regions were the frontal region (20.7%), the cheek region (16%) and the orbital region (15.5%), because they are exposed areas and are projected onto the skull, coupled with the fact that drivers neglect to wear protective equipment such as helmets and safety belts, and there is also the inadvertent consumption of alcoholic beverages by cyclists, which further favors the occurrence of accidents.

However, it has been shown that when a thorough assessment and proper management are carried out, facial injuries can be treated with sutures and dressings, favoring a good prognosis with the repair of injuries and minimization of sequelae.

REFERENCES

ALCANTARA, Alice et al. Evaluation of facial mimicry in children with facial burns. **Dermatofuncional uptodate,** online library. 2009.

AMERICAN COLLEGE OF SURGEONS COMMITTEE ON TRAUMA. Advanced Trauma Life Support - ATLS, 2004

BARRETO, Geraldine Rose de Andrade Borges et al. Facial burn: speech therapy approach in the prevention of microstomia. **Revista Brasileira de Queimaduras**, v. 10, n. 1, p. 35-38, 2011.

BOLT, R.W.; Watts, P.G. The relationship between a etiology and distribution of facial lacerations. **Injury** Extra, v. 35, n. 1, p. 6-11, 2004.

BRAZIL. Ministry of Health. National emergency care policy / Ministry of Health. - Brasilia: Ministry of Health, 2003. 228 p.: ill. - (Series E. Health Legislation)

CARVALHO, T.B.; Cancian, L.R.; Marques, C.G.; Piatto, V.B.; Maniglia, J.V.; Molina, F.D. Six years of facial trauma care: an epidemiological analysis of 355 cases. **Braz J Otorhinolaryngol**. Sep-Oct; v. 76, n. 5, p. 565-574, 2010.

CHAIA, A.; Nova, A.B.;Gaffre, G. Treatment of soft tissue injuries of the face.In: Associagao Brasileira de Odontologia; Pedrosa SF, Vasconcellos, R. J. H, Prado R, organizadores. PRO ODONTO CIRURGIA update program in surgical dentistry: Cycle 7. Porto alegre: Artmed panamericana;. P. 57-129. 2013

CLARK, N.; Birely, B.; Manson, P.N.; Slezak, S.; Kolk, C.V.; Robertson, B.High-energy ballistic and avulsive facial injuries: classification, patterns, and an algorithm for primary reconstruction. **Plast Reconstr Surg.** v. 98, n. 4, p. 583-601, 1996.

DANTAS, R.F.; Dias, M.A.P.; Dantas-Filho, M.O.; Ribeiro, E.D.; Andrade,

G.S.S. Soft tissue injury caused by a white weapon - literature review.
Rev. Odontol.Univ. Cid. Sao Paulo, v. 25, n. 1, p. 40-6, 2013

DE MACEDO, Jefferson Lessa Soares; DA SILVA, Adilson Alves. Primary closure of facial bites. **Revista do Colegio Brasileiro de Cirurgioes**, v. 27, n. 5, p. 316-320, 2018.

DIARIO DE PERNAMBUCO. Traffic accidents on federal highways cost

R$12.3 billion in

2014.(http://www.diariodepernambuco.com.br/brasil/capa_brasil/) 2014.

DORNELAS, Marilho Tadeu; FERREIRA, Ana Paula Rocha; CAZARIM, Daniele Barros. Treatment of burns in special areas. **HU Magazine**, v. 35, n. 2, 2009.

FONSECA, J. RAYMOND. **Oral and Maxillofacial Trauma** - 4ª Ed. Rio de Janeiro. Elsevier, 2015.

JAMES R. HUPP. **Contemporary Oral and Maxillofacial Surgery** - 6th Ed. Rio de Janeiro. Elsevier, 2015.

JARDIM, E.C.G.; Santiago junior, J.F.; Guastaldi, F.P.S. Facial Injuries: Case Report **Revista Odontologica de Aragatuba**, v.31, n.1, p. 73-77, Jan/Jun, 2010.

KRUG, E.G.; Sharma, G.K.; Lozano, L. The global burden of injuries. Am J Public Health, v. 90, n. 4, p. 523, 2000.

LEITE SEGUNDO, A.V, Gondim, D.G.A.; Caubi, A.F. Treatment of facial injuries. **Rev. Cir. Traumatol.** Camaragibe; v. 7, n. 1, p. 9-16, 2007.

MELO, R.E.V.A.; Vitor, C.M.A.; Silva, M.B.L.; Luna, L.A.; Firmo, A.C.B. Dentoalveolar trauma. **International journal of dentistry**, recife, v. 2, n. 2, p. 266-72, July/December 2003.

MIRANDA, Cristiana Ferreira Jardim de; SILVA, Jose Ailton da; MOREIRA, Elvio Carlos. Human rabies transmitted by dogs: risk areas in Minas Gerais,

Brazil, 1991-1999. **Cadernos de Saude Publica**, v. 19, p. 91-99, 2003.

NOGUEIRA NETO, J.N.; Muniz, V.R.V.M.; Figueiredo, L.M.G.; Freire, F.P.F.; Souza, A.S. Stab wound to the maxillofacial region: Case report Rev. **Cir. Traumatol. Buco-Maxilo-Fac.**, Camaragibe v.15, n.1, p. 41-44, jan./mar. 2015

WORLD HEALTH ORGANIZATION. Pan American Health Organization. Regional Strategic Plan. Geneva, 2007.

PETERSON, L.J. Peterson's principles of oral and maxillofacial surgery. 2 ed. London: BC DeckerInc Hamilton; 2004.

PRADO, ROBERTO. SALIN, MARTHA. **Oral and Maxillofacial Surgery - Diagnosis and Treatment -** 2ª Ed. Guanabara, 2018.

QUIRINO, L.C.; Paulesini Jr, W.; Masa, A.P.P.; Silva, J.P.; Sagara, G.T.P. Treatment of soft tissue injuries: clinical case reportRev. **odontol.UNESP,** vol.39, n. Especial , 2010.

ROSELINO, L.M.R.; Bregagnolo, L.A.; Pardinho, M.A.B.S.; Chiaperini, A.; Bergamo, A L.; De Santin, L. N.; Bregagnolo, J.C.;Watanabe ,M.G.C.; Silva, R.H.A. Oral and maxillofacial injuries in men from the Ribeirao Preto region (SP) between 1998 and 2002. **odontologia, ciencia e saude - revista do cromg**,v. 10, n. 2, p. 71-7, 2009 Apr/ Mai/ Jun 2009.

SANCHES, Simone; DUARTE, Sebastiao Junior Henrique; PONTES, Elenir Rose Jardim Cury. Characterization of victims of firearm injuries treated by the Mobile Emergency Care Service in Campo Grande, Mato Grosso do Sul. **Saude e Sociedade**, v. 18, p. 95-102, 2009.

SANTOS, J.S.; Kemp, R. Basic fundamentals for surgery and perioperative care. **Medicina (Ribeirao Preto. Online),** v. 44, n. 1, p. 2-17, jan/mar. 2011

SASTRY, S.M.; Sastry, C.M.; Paul, B.K.; Baim, L. Champion, H.R. Leading causes of facial trauma in the major trauma outcome study. **Plast. Reconstr. Surg.**, Baltimore, v.95, n.1, p.196-197, Jan.1995.

STATE HEALTH DEPARTMENT OF PERNAMBUCO. Analysis
Situational analysis of the IX Health Region of Pernambuco. Ouricuri, 2013.

SERRA, Alberto N. Bolgiani et al. Update on the local treatment of burns.
Revista Brasileira de Queimaduras, v. 9, n. 2, p. 38-44, 2010.

SHAIKH, Z.S.; Worrall, S.F. Epidemiology of facial trauma in a sample of
patients aged 1-18 years. **Injury,** v. 33, n. 8, p. 669-671, 2002.

SINGER, A.J.; Gulla, J.R.N.; Hein, M.P.A.; Marchini, S.P.A.; Chale, S.M.D.;
Arora, P.M.D. Single-layer versus double-layer closure of facial lacerations: a
randomized controlled trial. **Plasti. Reconstr. Surge,** Baltimore, v. 116, n. 2, p.
363-368, Aug. 2005.

SOUZA JUNIOR, E. F. D., MORAIS, H. H. A. D., LUCENA, E. E. D. S.,
CAVALCANTI, J. R. L. D. P., GUZEN, F. P., ARAUJO, D. P.. D., &
BARBALHO, J. C. M. State of the art in the treatment of mandibular fractures
caused by firearms: case report. **RGO-Revista Gaucha de Odontologia**, v. 66,
n. 1, p. 88-95, 2018.

TAHER, A.A. Management of weapon injuries to the craniofacial skeleton. **J
Craniofac Surg,** v. 9, n. 4, p. 371-382, Jul.1998.

TELES, Guilherme Gurgel do Amaral et al . Treatment of superficial second-
degree burns on the face and neck with topical heparin: a comparative,
prospective and randomized study. **Rev. Bras. Cir. Plast.,** Sao Paulo , v. 27, n.
3, p. 383-386, Sept. 2012

VALDERRAMA, L.S. Clinical application of povidone iodine oral antiseptic
1% (Betadineouthwash) and povidone-iodine skin antiseptic 10% (Betadine
solution) for the management ofodontogenic and deep fascial space infection.
Dermatology. v. 212, n. Suppl. 1, p. 112-114, 2006.

VIEIRA, C.L.; Araujo, D.C.C.; Ribeiro, M.L.S.; Laureano Filho, J.R.Soft tissue
injuries in patients victimized by oral and maxillofacial trauma. **Rev. Cir.
Traumatol.** Camaragibe v.13, n.1, p. 89-96, jan./mar. 2013

ZAVA, I.; Canonice, A.; Carvalho, B.M.; Zanetti, L.S.S.; Leal, M.P.S.; Salin, A.A. Prado, R.; Goncalves, S.L.M. Treatment of facial soft tissue wounds. Associagao Brasileira de Odontologia; Pedrosa SF, Vasconcellos, R. J. H, Prado R, organizers. PRO ODONTO CIRURGIA update program in surgical dentistry: Cycle 4. Porto Alegre: Artmed pan-americana; 2010. (system of continuing health education at a distance; v.1).

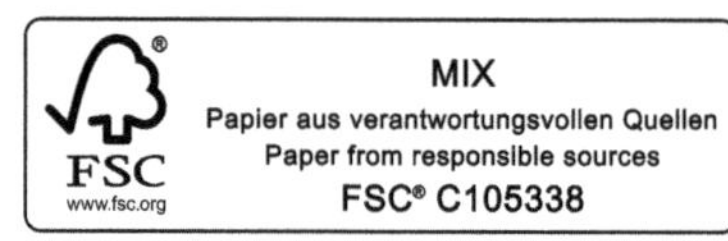

Printed by Books on Demand GmbH, Norderstedt / Germany